Distribution, publication, and copying in any form are prohibited and subject to damages.

TEN HYPNOSES

Copying, publishing, and sharing with third parties are only permitted with the written consent of the author. Please observe the notes on copyright and usage.

Distribution, publication, and copying in any form are prohibited and subject to damages.

Copying, publishing, and sharing with third parties are only permitted with the written consent of the author. Please observe the notes on copyright and usage.

Ingo Michael Simon

TEN HYPNOSES

29
FEAR OF HEIGHTS

Distribution, publication, and copying in any form are prohibited and subject to damages.

© 2024 Ingo Michael Simon
All rights reserved.
Independently published
www.ingosimon.com

Important Notes for Urgent Attention:

The contents of this book are based on the practical experiences of the author with hypnosis applications and psychotherapy in a trance state. Although the author has strived for the utmost care, errors or misunderstandings in the presentation cannot be completely excluded. Therapeutic work with people and the application of hypnosis are solely the responsibility of the hypnotist. It cannot be ruled out that parts of this book may be misunderstood or that the application of a presented procedure may cause an undesirable reaction in the client. The author also assumes no co-responsibility if work with a client is carried out with reference to the statements in this book.

The Author:

Ingo Michael Simon studied psychology and education and is a hypnotherapist with practices in southwestern Germany and Switzerland. With the help of hypnosis-supported psychotherapy, he primarily treats people with persistent psychological conditions. His practice focuses on anxiety disorders, pathological compulsions, and psychosomatic illnesses. His therapeutic offerings mainly include classical and modern hypnosis applications and the dreamland therapy he developed himself.

Copying, publishing, and sharing with third parties are only permitted with the written consent of the author. Please observe the notes on copyright and usage.

Distribution, publication, and copying in any form are prohibited and subject to damages.

INTRODUCTION	6
COPYRIGHT AND USAGE	8
HYPNOSIS 1	10
HYPNOSIS 2	15
HYPNOSIS 3	20
HYPNOSIS 4	26
HYPNOSIS 5	30
HYPNOSIS 6	35
HYPNOSIS 7	40
HYPNOSIS 8	45
HYPNOSIS 9	50
HYPNOSIS 10	55
ALL TITLES IN THE SERIES	60

Copying, publishing, and sharing with third parties are only permitted with the written consent of the author. Please observe the notes on copyright and usage.

Distribution, publication, and copying in any form are prohibited and subject to damages.

Introduction

The series "Ten Hypnoses" is very well known in Germany, Austria, and Switzerland as a collection of texts for therapeutic work and is used by numerous psychotherapeutic practices, doctors, therapists, coaches, and other helping professionals. I am pleased to now be able to offer these texts in other countries as well.

Most therapists have their own methods for inducing and deepening trance as well as for exiting trance. Therefore, I have focused on the main part of the hypnosis. The texts in this book can be integrated as the main part into any hypnosis process. The texts in this collection use various hypnosis techniques. I will not explain these in detail, as I assume that users have the appropriate training. It is also not necessary to understand the exact structure or functioning of the different parts. The texts can simply be read aloud, and they will have their effect.

Decide for yourself which text best suits your client or patient at any given time. You can also combine passages from different texts. It is not about using all ten hypnoses in sequence. It is a selection of possibilities.

Copying, publishing, and sharing with third parties are only permitted with the written consent of the author. Please observe the notes on copyright and usage.

I want to emphasize that books cannot replace therapy. Psychotherapy or other therapeutic treatments involve much more. A careful diagnosis is the necessary basis for deciding on the use of methods, including whether hypnosis or one of my texts should be used. Even in this case, preparatory discussions, follow-up discussions during the session, and of course, a therapeutic concept for the sequence of sessions and the content approaches are essential parts of therapy. This cannot and should not be achieved with a collection of texts.

In any case, I wish you much success in your work and I am pleased if my text templates can contribute in a small way.

Ingo Michael Simon

Copyright and Usage

Copying, publishing, and sharing with third parties is prohibited and only permitted with the written consent of the author. Please observe the following copyright and usage guidelines.

This work has been carefully crafted and created to the best of the author's knowledge and personal experience. It comprises text templates and application guidelines for professional hypnosis sessions. The author is a licensed psychotherapist with extensive experience in psychotherapy, coaching, and personal training using hypnotic techniques and methods. Nevertheless, the author and the publisher assume no liability for the accuracy of information, instructions, and advice, nor for any typographical errors. The author and publisher accept no responsibility or liability for the application of these texts and recommendations with clients or patients, nor for any potential consequences or unexpected reactions. It is expressly noted that the application of therapeutic and advisory techniques and formulations lies solely and entirely within the responsibility of the practitioner. This also applies to adherence to the boundaries of legally regulated medical and therapeutic practices. The fact that a book containing action proposals is freely available for sale does not imply that its application with clients or patients is permitted for everyone.

Hypnosis 1

You have decided to change your fear of heights today... ...To replace your previous fear of heights with calmness and security... ...You want to replace that feeling of fear... ...You've set this thought in your mind... ...and that's the right step, the right approach because our thoughts can indeed influence and control our experiences... ...So, you are fully focusing on the thought of truly overcoming your fear of heights... ...today already... ...It's truly remarkable how well you're able to make this thought very strong now... ...to place this goal of liberation right at the forefront... ...because nothing is more important now than freeing yourself from fear... ...nothing is more significant than achieving the freedom from fear that you are experiencing today... ...Every fiber of your body, every single cell is attuned to this... ...every thought follows this goal of liberation...

You know the burdensome thoughts of fear... ...Until now, just the thought of height, of a ladder or an open staircase, a glass elevator, or a balcony high up in a tall building, would give you an uncomfortable feeling... ...even before you actually went up... ...Today, you realize that it was primarily these thoughts that produced the fear... ...these anticipatory thoughts that allowed nothing else but fear... ...but today, your thoughts are changing, and this is possible because you now know and focus entirely on the fact that thoughts influence your feelings... ...so, a good and strong thought can help you too... ...Today, you are creating a strong thought, one that is stronger than fear... ...a thought that takes precedence and becomes the most important thought... ...It is the thought... ...The higher I go, the bigger and stronger I become... ...This is a good thought because it helps you... ...It becomes the truth, just as your anticipatory thoughts became truth in the past... ...Your anticipatory thought is... ...The higher I go, the bigger and stronger I become... ...Good... ...very good... ...That's right...

Your body also reacts to your thoughts, you know this... ...to fearful thoughts, the body responds with tension, and to freedom, the body responds with calmness and relaxation... ...and that's what you can feel right now, very clearly... ...You are calm and relaxed... ...very calm and very relaxed... ...and your new thought relaxes your body even more, making tension completely impossible... ...The thought... ...The higher I go, the bigger and stronger I become... ...brings your body to rest, and a calm body makes fear impossible... ...You can even test this now, because now you can imagine height and still remain calm... ...You could now, in your mind, stand high up on a skyscraper, and yet you remain calm because your body helps you with this... ...Your body now and always helps you stay calm and composed... ...especially at heights...

Body and mind form a unit, always... ...Just as your body feels, so do your emotions... ...and your moods and emotions also affect your body... ...and now the calmness and relaxation of your body affect your mood... ...because everything within you is calm and becomes even calmer and more comfortable... ...your feelings align with the trance of your body... ...and deep within you, this new connection between calmness and height emerges... ...pleasant calmness and pleasant height... ...and the higher you go, the higher your calmness also rises... ...the further you go up, the more intense the feeling of calmness becomes... ...This new connection between calmness and height becomes so firm and stable that you can feel it clearly in your waking life... ...with every step on an open staircase or a ladder, you feel the connection between calmness and height... ...with every thought of height, you feel the new and stable connection of calmness and height within you...

So, it becomes second nature to face height because you are now strong enough for it... ...You are now stronger than the height... ...and stronger than any fear... ...You take on this special challenge of height, embrace it with a sporting spirit and joy... ...You approach the height... ...In the past, you often tried to avoid height because you mentally prepared yourself for fear, but today it's completely different... ...From now on, you embrace height as a challenge that you are sure to master... ...You approach height and know very well that your new thought is with you... ...The higher I go, the bigger and stronger I become... ...You approach height and know very well that the new and stable connection between calmness and height makes it easy for you to ascend and feel comfortable high up... ...high up, there you are... ...high up, there you are... ...You are absolutely certain that your thoughts help you control your body and your feelings because it has always been so...

…just as it was with fear… …and today, security takes the place of fear… …Now…

You have taken on your goal today, have faced your former fear of heights… …and it was easier than you thought because it is the thoughts that decide everything… …and you have a new thought, a thought that has now become the most important of all… …Your thought is… …The higher I go, the bigger and stronger I become… …and this new thought puts you in an inner calmness that your body can feel… …Your body relaxes at the thought of height, and your body also calms your feelings, giving you the feeling of calmness and security… …and letting you become calm inside… …Calmness and height are firmly connected… …Calmness and height are one… …Calmness and height are truly one… …therefore, you approach every height with composure, see it as a challenge that you are truly capable of meeting… … …high up, there you are… …high up, there you are…

Hypnosis 2

You have a goal... ...You want to overcome the fear of heights, to be able to stand on a ladder or a balcony high up and feel good about it... ...Your goal is: I will overcome my fear of heights... ...You are now preparing to achieve this goal... ...to achieve good success today already... ...You are now more focused than ever on overcoming your fear of heights... ...to achieve more today than you thought possible... ...Today, you are absolutely and completely focused on your goal of conquering your fear of heights... ...because you want to achieve the greatest success today... ...maybe even leave the fear of heights behind completely... ...It's truly remarkable how well you can focus on your goal today... ...and even more remarkable is that you are facing this fear today, ready to confront it... ...to let it be there and deal with it, to take away its power... ...but the most important and greatest thing is that today you are taking control... ...today you are taking control... ...You are more powerful than fear...

First, focus on your strengths, and I'm sure you have them... ...Simply focus now on your feelings and also on your bodily sensations because by doing so, you automatically connect with your own power and strength... ...Often, your strength has helped you get through difficult situations and gain the upper hand in tough situations... ...it works today as well... ...You are strong, and your strength is now becoming clearer... ...slowly entering your feelings... ...You are truly very strong, and you are now awakening this great strength within you... ...because strength helps you significantly in overcoming fear... ...You are stronger today than ever before, much stronger than ever before... ...and you can use this special power today to truly overcome your fear at heights... ...You are stronger than the height... ...you are much stronger than the height... ...You have the power...

Today, you are working on a new mindset and a new feeling... ...Being high up is the theme... ...being in the height... ...or going up high... ...In the height, everything is fine... ...high up, everything is okay... ...You tell yourself this and accept this thought... ...Height is truly indifferent to you; you don't even think about it... ...high up, everything is unimportant... ...high up, many things are completely irrelevant... ...You accept this thought and let it work deep within you... ...In the height, there is no more fear... ...high up, fear disappears... ...high up, fear truly disappears... ...This thought is powerful, and you are just as powerful... ...you can turn it into a belief... ...you can do it now... ...you can even do it very quickly... ...it happens faster than you think, and fear can go away...

When you stand high up, you can even feel freer and better than when you're down on the ground... ...because up there, you can feel a sense of lightness... ...Up high, you can rise above things... ...on a ladder, you can see further than from the ground... ...so you can feel freer and also stronger because you have the overview... ...On a high ladder, it is even better for you because there, you can breathe more freely and deeply... ...and see much further, really take in everything... ...so you can feel comfortable and gain something really good from the height... ...On a very high ladder, you feel the best because you are still up there after the fear has already disappeared... ...high up, you feel free and strong... ...high up, you feel truly free and truly strong... ...high up, you feel completely free and absolutely strong... ...from today on, it is so... ...exactly like that... ...just like now in trance...

You have taken a big step... ...You have overcome your fear of heights with your thoughts... ...and what is possible in thought is also possible with and through thoughts... ...You have reached an important milestone and become stronger than fear... ...today is that special day when you accomplished this... ...You have taken a very important step by becoming significantly stronger than fear... ...today, you did this excellently... ...you made yourself bigger and stronger than your previous fear of or in height... ...Today, you achieved the greatest possible step because today you have already changed your inner attitude towards height... ...Height can be insignificant and unimportant... ...it can be irrelevant to you... ...But height can also be positive because in a strong position up there, you become even more powerful... ...You have succeeded... ...You have control over your fear of heights and can continue to have control over it... ...Soon, you will be able to laugh about it because you can no longer feel it... ...because it has disappeared, and you feel comfortable high up... ...just as comfortable as on the ground... ...You can be proud of yourself for overcoming your fear of heights... ...for achieving it today... ...You can be very proud of yourself, and you have every reason to be because today, you succeeded in overcoming your old fear of heights... ...You can be prouder of yourself today than ever before because you have truly achieved this inner liberation... ...you have conquered the fear...

Today, you have earned your freedom... ...and this freedom will remain with you... ...because everything you achieve in your imagination, you also achieve later in your waking life... ...you can experience there how you handle height well... ...how you still feel good when you climb... ...You can test it in your everyday life because you can really experience there how you handle height with ease and how height no longer bothers you... ...how you even feel comfortable when climbing... ...You have really succeeded, and every day, your fear of heights becomes a thing of the past... ...a past that lies far behind... ...Fear was yesterday; from today on, you have power... ...from today on, you truly have power...

Hypnosis 3

Anchor Technique (Visual Anchor, Post-Hypnotic)

An anchor (or trigger) is a stimulus that is meant to create a specific feeling or evoke a particular thought. It serves as a signal that the client perceives, which then triggers an internal process. The established anchor then replaces the suggestion. In everyday life, a client can use an anchor to trigger or establish a desired state without being in a trance. Various stimuli can be used as anchors/triggers. I work with the following options, which I also use in the series "Ten Hypnoses": physical anchors (clenching a hand, pressing the base of the thumb...), visual anchors (symbols, word cards...), acoustic anchors (signal sounds like a phone ring, melodies...), olfactory anchors (scented oils...), haptic anchors (comfort objects, talismans...). I also distinguish between peri-hypnotic and post-hypnotic anchors. Peri-hypnotic anchors are those primarily used during hypnosis, where the therapist sets up the anchor and then repeatedly triggers it as a supplement to suggestions and visualizations.

Post-hypnotic anchors are primarily set up for the time after the session so that the client can help themselves with it.

Today, we want to place an anchor... ...an anchor is a simple tool that helps you let go of the fear of heights and stay free from it... ...like an anchor that holds a ship in place so that it remains steady in a storm and high waves, your anchor will help you stay in control and always maintain control over the situation... ...especially when you go up or stand high above... ...And you should always be able to carry your anchor with you... ...first, it should help you stay calm or become calm when fear could arise... ...and then it should constantly ensure that fear can no longer arise because you simply carry your anchor with you... ...You have this goal of getting rid of your fear of heights, and with that, you have a target thought that tells you... ...I feel comfortable even high up... ...You want to firmly anchor this thought to avoid falling into the trap of fear of heights when you go somewhere high...

[Keep a small card ready with the inscription "I feel comfortable even high up" and discuss with the client before hypnosis that you will hand them the card during the session. There is no need to open their eyes for this. Simply announce a touch again shortly before handing over the card and touch the client's hand with it so they can grasp it afterward. Just follow the instructions in the text!]...

But first, you need to be free of fear... ...free of fear now, in this moment... ...That's likely very easy; you probably have no fear at this moment, after all, you're in a trance and quite relaxed... ...and in relaxation, fear cannot exist... ...only one of the two can be present... ...Relaxation or fear... ...and now you feel relaxation... ...only relaxation... ...Now you feel the relaxation even more clearly... ...and in the state of relaxation, you feel free from fear of heights... ...and very light inside... ...the more you manage to focus on yourself right now, on the feeling of relaxation... ...in this very moment... ...the better you can now also feel that fear of heights is not present at all, not present at all right now... ...Now you don't have to worry about anything... ...now you don't have to accomplish anything... ...now you have peace...

Now, in deep relaxation, you can encounter yourself free of fear, simply let go of all fearful thoughts, and feel free...

...It's much easier now than usual... ...You accept yourself at this moment and are free from fear... ...The more clearly you can feel the relaxation now, the better you can also feel free... ...So feel the relaxation and accept yourself without fear... ...Now... ...Now it's happening... ...You can feel calmness and experience and accept yourself without fear... ...Now, I'm placing the card in your hand... ...

[Touch the client's hand and hand them the card. They can keep their eyes closed.]...

...Feel the card in your hand... ...You know what it says... ...It says: I feel comfortable even high up... ...You think about this sentence, this attitude... ...You feel that you feel good right now... ...You are completely free from fear now and feel good... ...and now you focus on yourself... ...resolve, as it says on the card, to feel comfortable even high up... ...to not let fear arise anymore... ...The card reminds you that you can feel comfortable, just as you feel comfortable now, because it's always and everywhere possible... ...especially when going up... ...The card helps you because whenever you carry it with you, you feel as secure as you do now... ...when you carry it with you, you feel as good as you do now because it reminds you of how good you feel now... ...your whole body remembers, your entire being remembers the relaxation and stays relaxed... ...your anchor helps you with this... ...You know that you can always free yourself from fear... ...just like today... ...the card helps you with that... ...This card in your hand is your anchor... ...the anchor that keeps you grounded in calmness... ...the anchor that prevents you from drifting into fear... ...You don't go into fear; you stay in safety... ...you stay in exactly this safe feeling that you feel now because your anchor holds you there... ...Your anchor keeps you safe...

You can carry the card with you every day... ...and whenever you feel like fear of heights might catch up with you or ensnare you, you can take it in your hand and read what it says... ...I feel comfortable even high up... ...and immediately you feel more calmness and a sense of freedom deep inside... ...just like now... ...exactly like now... ...Also, whenever even a single thought of fear could arise or the idea that fear could return at some point, simply take the card in your hand, look at it consciously and deliberately, and read what it says... ...I feel comfortable even high up... ...and immediately you feel more calmness and a sense of freedom deep inside... ...with just one look at the card... ...even when you hold the card in your hand or touch it without reading it, you feel the release from the fear of heights clearly... ...just like today... ...every day, just like today...

Hypnosis 4

Height should become pleasant, that's your goal... ...The time of fear is coming to an end now; it should be over... ...You've had this goal for a long time, but today more than ever... ...Today, you want more than ever to make height something bearable... ...and even more than that... ...You want to make height something that is pleasant... ...because you want to feel free... ...You want to feel free when going up... ...You want to feel free when you are high up... ...Freedom and you, way up high... ...Freedom and you, way up high... ...That's why you're here today... ...that's why you're going deeper into trance and preparing yourself to turn your goal into an inner conviction today... ...because once you've succeeded in turning your goal into a deep inner conviction, you'll feel truly free... ...truly free... ...high up and deep within... ...high up and deep within...

We begin... ...First, it's important to let go of distracting thoughts, and this is quite simple when you focus on an image... ...Imagine sitting in a pillar of light... ...a column of white light, and you are sitting calmly in the middle... ...You look at the light wall surrounding you, it's all around you and shines pleasantly... ...So you only see the white light around you and find a pleasant stillness within you... ...All thoughts drift away... ...It's as if all your thoughts are drawn to and dissolved by the white light, and you simply allow yourself to rest in the white light... ...You only see white light that shines through your skin into your body and completely floods you inside... ...White light flows through your body, making you feel light...

Then, the pillar of light slowly expands, becomes bigger and wider... ...The space in the light becomes wider and more open... ...The pillar of light becomes bigger and wider, and you are always exactly in the middle because that's where there's the most calm... ...there, you can rest and simply be, because that's enough... ...Being here is really enough... ...and on the wall of white light, writing gradually appears... ...a script that you can now clearly read... ...it says...

High up is my greatest freedom, high up, I feel good.

... [Read the affirmation slowly and a little louder than the previous text to emphasize it. Then pause for about 30 seconds before continuing to read.]...

This phrase now unfolds its effect deep within you... ...because when there is only white light around you, and you are in the middle, a good and helpful phrase or slogan becomes your deep belief... ...if this phrase aligns with your goals... ...and you have this goal... ...This affirmation, this belief, will become true whenever it aligns with your desires... ...and you have the desire to experience freedom at heights... ...to feel good high up... ...so this special phrase becomes a new and deep belief...

This new belief becomes your deep conviction today... ...a conviction that you can repeat and use like an inner creed... ...like a commitment to your belief in yourself...

High up is my greatest freedom, high up, I feel good.

... ...Now, take a deep breath... ...Let your breath flow consciously into your body and follow its path... ...Feel how you take in this fresh air and how it fills your body... ...and with this breath, you also take in your affirmation... ...with each subsequent breath, it's as if you inhale your affirmation, your belief and let it flow deep into you... ...your breath anchors this attitude, which is already becoming an inner conviction... ...a conviction of your emotional world, which is completely attuned to the freedom of height...

Excellent, truly excellent, because it's accomplished... ...this new attitude is now your own... ...it is firmly anchored and available to you at any time... ...As soon as you experience a situation involving height in your waking life that used to be difficult, your subconscious now immediately provides you with the feeling of freedom, and you automatically adjust to the fact that freedom grows with every step upward... ...greater freedom with every step up... ...and if you want to intensify the effect so that fear can't even arise, not even as a thought, just tell yourself consciously and deliberately... ...High up is my greatest freedom, high up, I feel good... ...and immediately your entire being shifts into a calm state that you can clearly feel... ...You've done it... ...you've succeeded, and with that, you succeed every day anew... ...every day, freedom in height... ...every day, freedom high up... ...Freedom and you... ...Freedom and you...

Hypnosis 5

You have made a decision... ...The fear of heights should go; it should be over once and for all... ...You've already tried to end it, but in the past, it was stronger... ...but even the fear of heights was a part of you... ...and if it was a part of you, then its strength and stubbornness came from you... ...like a misdirected force that you correct today... ...Today, you use this strength and your own stubbornness to insist that the fear disappears... ...You end the fear of heights... ...You truly end it... ...Today, you think about whether your fear really has to do with height... ...you ask yourself where it actually comes from... ...Whatever may have happened, often things are different than we believe... ...because often a fear of heights or fear at heights shows up, but actually, it's about another fear or a completely different feeling... ...and most of the time, it's about your own feelings being suppressed too often... ...maybe not being allowed because they were once forbidden... ...or you often thought you had to deal with your feelings alone to spare others or for a reason only you know...

Maybe you've thought so far that you can feel your emotions well... ...because, for example, you felt the fear of heights so clearly... ...but there might also be suppressed feelings that you no longer feel so clearly... ...because fear was often at the forefront, or because you were too often preoccupied with other things you felt responsible for... ...Then you could take care of yourself less, less of your true feelings... ...and when we keep our feelings inside too long and deal with them ourselves, it creates an overpressure within us that does something... ...It can make us sick or produce a special fear... ...for you, it was the fear of heights... ...Imagine for a moment that your feelings were like balloons... ...and each balloon represents a feeling... ...and because feelings want to come out, these balloons are filled with a very light gas... ...with helium... ...They would immediately fly up, rise into the sky and be very light there, if they weren't being held down... ...But today, it's about the deep feelings that you have often suppressed, probably had to suppress, because you couldn't deal with them any other way... ...So many of your feeling balloons are tied to a heavy stone that holds them down... ...Imagine many of your feeling balloons tied to a heavy stone, to a heavy stumbling block... ...and the balloons want to go up, to free themselves...

Now imagine how it often was when the fear of heights suddenly appeared... ...Deep inside you, there were these balloons that you now imagine before your inner eye... ...They wanted to go up, to the surface and beyond, because they wanted to be seen and felt... ...The balloons of your feelings wanted to rise high... ...but something in you didn't allow that... ...Something in you produced this fear that kept you on the ground and kept your feelings small... ...That's just how it happened, you didn't do anything wrong... ...You didn't have control over it, but today you do... ...There are many feelings in you that want to come out, and over time, you will free them all... ...a very special feeling is particularly connected to the fear of heights, a feeling you've wanted to let out for a long time... ...maybe a difficult or burdensome or even a beautiful feeling that you couldn't show before... ...This feeling has also been tied to the heavy stumbling block for years... ...maybe because you thought it was a bad or inappropriate feeling... ...but there's no such thing... ...Actions can be bad, but feelings cannot...

Images and pictures in us are always a reflection of what is possible deep in our emotions... ...and today it's possible to free a large part of your suppressed feelings... ...finally letting them rise high so that they become free and light at great heights... ...So now you imagine that you cut the strings holding the feeling balloons back, thereby freeing the balloons of feelings... ...One by one, you untie them... ...and immediately the feeling balloons rise high... ...They fly high into the sky, and you watch them... ...The balloons of freed feelings fly high into freedom... ...they rise higher and higher... ...and feel free... ...Watch them as they rise... ...a lot of freed balloons... ...a lot of freed feelings... ...Balloons of old hurts fly high and feel free... ...Balloons of anger fly high and feel free... ...Balloons of disappointments fly high and feel free... ...A very special feeling that you've always wanted to let out rises very high and feels free... ...infinitely free... ...All feelings rise high and feel freed... ...You can see them, and you can feel that feelings rise high... ...Let them be because none of your feelings can be wrong... ...All feelings rise high and are free... ...and fear fades... ...Fear fades, and in its place comes freedom... ...Freedom within you...

Today, you realized that it's good to let your feelings rise high every day, like unrestrained gas balloons that want to be free high up... ...Your deep inner self is fully attuned to letting your feelings rise high every day, so high that you can clearly feel and see them... ...because rising feelings help you feel free... ...You acknowledge your feelings and accept them as your true feelings... ...so they rise high and are freed and light... ...and whenever you go up, whenever you yourself rise high, you feel this liberation... ...you feel that you yourself feel free because your deep feelings are already free... ...and if you want to feel even lighter, simply imagine the fear itself as a big red balloon flying into the sky and bursting...

Hypnosis 6

This is the goal of the day: End of fear of heights... ...This fear has outlived its usefulness; it should go away today... ...it should become smaller, very small and insignificant... ...The fear of heights should go so that you can finally feel free again, free even and especially high up... ...The thought of going up or standing high above should leave you cold... ...The thought of being high up and looking down should be indifferent to you... ...Height should be indifferent and remain indifferent... ...That's your goal... ...That's the goal of the day... ...the most important goal, and exactly this goal is to be achieved... ...It can be achieved today; it is indeed possible... ...today already... ...Be free from fear today and remain free from fear...

Deep within you, in your feelings, there is a very special place... ...It is a place where an encounter is possible that will help you let go of the fear of heights... ...an encounter with yourself... ...or rather, with a part of yourself... ...a special part of yourself... ...This place is a place of freedom and lies where your mind cannot go in a waking state...

...but in trance, it is possible... ...here and today, it is possible... ...because you are in this special state of calm, where you can really look deep inside and see and find everything that belongs to you... ...Imagine that you could sink into your feelings... ...sink into yourself... ...deeper and deeper... ...a bit like falling into a deep sleep and beginning to dream... ...in a deep, deep sleep simply dreaming... ...and in your dream, you go to this place of inner encounter... ...You arrive at the place of inner encounter now...

You feel the presence of a person who is with you... ...You feel this presence in your feelings... ...There is someone with you, and you have the feeling that this person is very similar to you... ...It is dark around you, and you feel good... ...You feel safe and secure because this special place is a place of security... ...It lies within you, and inside you, you are truly safe... ...Then you feel your hand being grasped... ...and it feels as if a very familiar hand is reaching for your hand... ...and slowly it becomes brighter at the place of encounter, and you can recognize the person who is with you and holding your hand to help you... ...It is yourself, standing there like a twin brother/twin sister [Please adjust to the client's gender]... ...facing you... ...Your alter ego extends its hand to you, holds your hand tightly to show you that you are not alone... ...that you are always protected and supported... ...protected and supported by yourself... ...because there are also strong parts within you that are without fear...

This part of you, which meets you here within, knows your fear... ...This helper/This helper within you is only here to help you... ...to help you experience height as normal again... ...with a feeling of security and strength... ...Understanding has often been lacking for you... ...You have experienced that many people could not or would not understand that you felt this fear so strongly... ...so you were often alone with your fear... ...you then doubted yourself and thought that you should be stronger or that something was wrong with you... ...But you are normal... ...You just have fear at heights, but you are normal... ...and your helper, this helping part, knows that... ...and this helper in you also knows that there are causes and reasons for this fear... ...often the development of a fear is very complex, and the causes are difficult to describe because there were so many moments and events that worked together until the fear could finally develop... ...but your helper is with you today to show you that it can be different... ...to extend a helping hand to you and make the fear smaller... ...and deep inside, you feel connected and safe... ...connected and safe... ...and with each breath, you feel a little freer... ...because your fear of heights is being absorbed by your helper... ...Every memory of fear, every fear you once had in the height or in connection with height or at the thought of height, flows from within you through your hand to the hand of your helper, who gladly accepts this fear... ...Your helper is a part of you... ...and so your fear of heights flows to a special part of you... ...to a part within you that can work on the fear there... ...so deep inside that the fear cannot be felt by your mind... ...Your helper can slowly dissolve this old fear inside by gradually working on and resolving the causes and background... ...deep inside, in the unconscious, that is completely sufficient... ...and as a result, you have more freedom... ...You, on the outside, in your waking life, have more freedom and feel good... ...You hand over your fear of heights to yourself, but you hand it over to a part within you... ...a part that can work on this fear very well because in the subconscious, this processing is possible... ...Until now, the fear was completely on the outside, burdening and disturbing you in everyday life... ...now you are deliberately giving it inside, because there it can be resolved... ...Your helper is this inner part that takes the fear with it and can work on and resolve it deep inside... ...That really works, it succeeds when you hand over all fearful thoughts... ...They now flow from your hand to the helping hand...

Everything happens on its own now... ...Your fear of heights flows more and more inward, so you no longer feel it... ...and inside, it can now be resolved, step by step, you can count on that... ...It will happen, your inner helper will take care of that for you... ...and you slowly return to the outside... ...from hand to hand, you stay connected to your inner helper and come back to the outside...

Hypnosis 7

You have decided to replace the fear of heights... ...You want to replace it with feelings and abilities you had before, in a time long before the fear of heights, because it wasn't always there... ...There was a time when you didn't even think about something like fear of heights or fear at heights... ...because it simply didn't exist... ...You had no fear; it only developed later... ...maybe you know why, or it's completely unclear... ...The good thing is that you don't have to know the causes to replace the fear... ...You just have to know the way to replace it... ...have to know how or where you can do it... ...Imagine you could feel like you used to when there was no fear of heights... ...If you imagine it, it's like a journey into the past... ...that's the journey we want to take together today because there you will find everything you need to replace the fear of heights today with your own potential... ...Potential that helps you be free from fear, just like you used to be...

Now go on an inner journey... ...a journey through the timeline of your life... ...through the images of your memory and the feelings of your life... ...maybe you remember many events in your life well, and it's like a movie running backward... ...or it's like a journey through a long tunnel that goes so fast it feels like flying or a train ride, and you simply let yourself drift... ...back to a time when fear of heights was not an issue yet... ...There was this time before fear of heights... ...It wasn't always there... ...There was a time when you didn't even think about the possibility of fear of heights because you felt secure... ...and on your journey, you get closer and closer to this time... ...It's as if you skip over the time of fear of heights... ...It's as if you jump back to a fear-free time... ...You don't have to make an effort for this; you don't have to do anything special or come up with something... ...no special memory in your thoughts... ...Simply imagine that you arrive in the time before fear of heights... ...in a time when there was still calmness and ease within you... ...even and especially when something involved height... ...even and especially when you yourself were involved with height... ...had to climb a ladder or wanted to... ...had to climb an open staircase or wanted to... ...It was easy back then... ...and that's where you arrive now...

Now stay in this earlier time... ...feel once more the life feeling of that time... ...the fearlessness and, with it, self-confidence and strength... ...That was normal for you back then... ...Self-confidence and strength... ...That was completely normal and natural... ...First, look around in your memory... ...See where you are... ...in what time of your life... ...Check how old you were when everything was still good... ...when you were still fearless... ...Look where you are, where your journey has taken you... ...and then fully immerse yourself in these images... ...or in the thought of really having arrived in this fear-free past... ...and fully enter the feeling of certainty that you are really there, in the fear-free time... ...You are in your thoughts back in the fear-free time... ...You are with inner images, with images before your inner eye, back in the fear-free time... ...You are with your feelings back in the fear-free time... ...and the good and strong feelings from back then come alive... ...It's your old self-confidence that is coming back... ...You feel your self-confidence inside you... ...It is coming back to life and becoming strong... ...a lively and strong self-confidence... ...Your old courage is being activated again... ...You feel this old courage becoming stronger... ...Your courage... ...It's your courage because you had this courage back then and have it today... ...Your old courage is becoming strong and stronger... ...Self-confidence and courage within you... ...Self-confidence and courage from you for you... ...and there are other strengths... ...another strong and helpful feeling is now coming alive within you... ...a feeling that was strong back then and is now coming back to life... ...a feeling or ability that helps you overcome the fear of heights... ...an ability that prevented fear back then is now awakening and blocking any possible fear now... ...Your strengths are becoming active, and they imprint themselves firmly within you so that you can use them anytime and always...

It's as if you could suddenly grasp and hold onto self-confidence, courage, and other strengths... ...You can actually hold onto them... ...feel them and firmly anchor them within you... ...You feel these helpful feelings in your body, so you can take them with you... ...and filled with your strengths, which are stronger than any fear, you go back on a journey... ...You take a journey into the future... ...It's as if you travel through a time tunnel from the past toward the future... ...filled with your strengths and completely free from fear, you travel to the present and beyond the present into the future... ...into a fear-free future... ...maybe a few months ahead... ...and there you stop, in a fear-free, near future... ...In this fear-free future, you have no fear of heights; it is no longer possible there... ...You look at how it is to climb a high ladder, ascend a high and open staircase, or experience a situation that was fearful in the past and is now easy... ...In this future, you feel your self-confidence and strength... ...You feel your potential, which safely and easily leads you upward... ...You at the top and strong... ...You at the top and strong...

Filled with this strength, with your courage, you can now calmly return to the present... ...to finally enjoy your own strength in the present, in your waking life... ...to experience in your present that you have this courage... ...that you can feel comfortable at the top... ...that you have overcome the fear with your own strength... ...The strength that was once within you and is still there today helps you... ...Your strength makes you free... ...free every day...

Hypnosis 8

Ideomotor Response

Ideomotor response refers to the phenomenon that our body follows our feelings and thoughts with movements. In everyday life, this following manifests as body posture, muscle tension, and movement patterns of a person, which naturally change with mood and thoughts. In trance, ideomotor signals can be used to receive information that the client cannot actively communicate. For example, the subconscious can answer questions with a pre-agreed finger signal. Of course, ideomotor responses can also be used suggestively, such as with arm levitations and catalepsies. An ideomotor approach strengthens trust in hypnosis and in one's ability to change, thus promoting therapy.

You want to erase the fear of heights today so that you can confidently go up... ...climb ladders, stairs, go onto a balcony, or climb a lookout tower... ...You want to decide again for yourself whether and when you go up... ...you want to regain and keep control over your life... ...You want to be self-determined and strong again... ...want to experience height calmly and securely... ...That's why you are here... ...You are here to achieve just that... ...here and today... ...once and for all... ...To do this, I invite your subconscious to work with me and with you... ...Your subconscious can and will help you... ...here and today... ...once and for all...

Imagine for a moment that your subconscious could make your arm feel light... ...so light that your arm rises into the air as if weightless... ...If your subconscious can do that, then it can also banish the fear of heights for you or make it light and build a feeling of security... ...but your subconscious can do even more... ...It can show you that it really does that, that it truly ends your fear of heights... ...because only then will your arm really become light... ...Your arm will become light and rise by itself, rise lightly upward as soon as your subconscious lets go of the fear of heights... ...So, imagine your right arm being very light, feather-light because three thick balloons are tied to it, filled with helium, and helium is a very light gas... ...Three thick helium balloons are tied to your right arm and pull your arm upward, and it follows the balloons that rise into the sky... ...as soon as your subconscious lets go of the fear of heights and it does so now... ...Your subconscious lets go, and your arm becomes lighter and rises upward... ...More helium balloons join in, and all are tied to your wrist... ...ten balloons pull your right arm... ...then twenty balloons that pull and pull on your right arm... ...Your arm is pulled upward, into the air... ...Your arm rises into the air... ...Your arm rises higher and higher, becoming feather-light... ...Your arm becomes light and rises into the air, rises into the air... ...Your arm rises higher and higher... ...Your arm becomes light like your thoughts and rises, rises into the air on its own...

[Please stay with it. The suggestive connection between the rising arm and letting go of fear has already been established. The continuous suggestion for the arm to rise will eventually lead to the arm rising, which will have the effect of reducing fear. Keep repeating the lightness and balloon suggestions until the arm moves – it will happen!]

... ...There you go... ...it works... ...your arm is floating in the air, and the helium balloons are holding it up... ...your arm is held in this exact position, and that is quite easy...

...Your arm remains in the air, and that's good... ...Simply open your eyes briefly; your arm will remain in this position... ...Open your eyes and look at your arm; it remains held in this position...

[Always have the client briefly look at the levitating arm during arm levitations, otherwise, it could be perceived as an illusion. It's important that the levitating arm is consciously experienced, as this strengthens the belief in and trust in the possibilities of hypnosis. No worries – the arm will continue to be held. No need for elaborate fractionations.]

Now, you can close your eyes again... ...Your arm is held up, has risen into the air, and is held there and becomes stiff like an iron rod... ...Your arm becomes very firm and stable, very firm and stable... ...Now your arm becomes firmer and remains here in the air, completely on its own... ...That's easy... ...it happens on its own... ...Your arm becomes firmer and completely immobile... ...nothing and no one could move your arm now... ...I'll show you by pressing against your arm, and it won't budge... ...Your arm is firm like an iron rod... ...very firm and stable...

[Press against the arm, which will offer significant resistance. The client experiences that their arm is truly cataleptic. But don't overdo it, please! Gentle pressure! The connection between catalepsy and new strength has already been established suggestively. The cataleptic arm "proves" to the client the inner change.]

… …It has worked; your arm has risen, and it holds firm… …I have told your subconscious that it should only allow this if it also erases the fear of heights so that you can also go up… …rise into the air, and that is what has happened…

You have achieved a lot now… …now the helium balloons may disappear, and your arm can become heavier again… …your arm becomes heavy again and slowly sinks onto the surface… …your fear of heights has been erased; that's the only reason your arm moved up, the only reason it rose into the air… …and now your arm can rest… …Your arm sinks back onto the surface and becomes completely relaxed… …Your arm is completely relaxed, and you have full control over your arm… …you can move it, and your fingers… …[Stay with it until the arm relaxes on the surface.]… …good… …very good… …The fear of heights is gone…

Hypnosis 9

You want to overcome your fear of heights today... ...want to change your feelings when you're up high... ...You've made a really good decision because, strictly speaking, you've never been afraid of heights or of being up high... ...It just showed up there... ...but that's not the same... ...Your fear developed at some point but wasn't really about height... ...that's often the case when we have problems... ...They show up in a different context, and we don't understand them anymore... ...Today, we're taking a journey back to the origin, and maybe you're wondering where the fear of heights really comes from and are already excited... ...or you're just looking forward to being able to erase the fear of heights on an inner journey... ...maybe you're looking forward to the fact that changing your perspective on and in the past can also positively change your experience today... ...Once you learned to be afraid, today you'll learn liberation...

Now your deep inner self goes on a journey through space and time... ...back to a time when the fear of heights did not exist yet... ...There was this time before the fear of heights... ...You can remember it... ...There was a time when you didn't think about the possibility that height could frighten you... ...and deep in your feelings, you are now going step by step back to this time... ...maybe not even that far back, just a few months or years... ...or this journey goes very far back... ...perhaps many years... ...and if you don't know exactly when it all started, just go very far back... ...back to your childhood, and if necessary, go back to the day you were born... ...For this, you don't have to do anything special, you don't need a specific memory in your mind... ...Simply imagine that you are inwardly going to the time before the fear... ...to a time when there was still a feeling of trust and security within you... ...so much trust and so much security that even height was completely okay... ...when height was completely okay... ...You arrive at this time now... ...You are in a time before the fear... ...You are in a time long before the fear of heights... ...in safety and trust... ...in a time of safety and trust...

And now you move forward in time... ...You are in your past, you are before the fear of heights, and time slowly moves forward... ...You approach the moment of the triggering situation, the moment when the fear of heights developed... ...maybe this journey is accompanied by images, and you actually remember... ...you approach a situation that triggered your fear of heights... ...maybe you already knew that it was this particular situation... ...or you are surprised that you are getting closer to this time or this specific situation... ...Whatever it is and wherever this journey takes you... ...whenever this time may have been... ...You now arrive at the moment of the trigger... ...in the moment when it all began, when your fear of heights was born, but you feel good now...

If you have visual memories, look at them, because you are doing well... ...If you don't have images, simply feel deep into your feelings, because it's the feeling of that time... ...but it felt different than fear of heights... ...because it wasn't really the height that scared you... ...it was the feeling of being alone... ...helpless and defenseless... ...and if the triggering situation did have to do with height, it wasn't really the height, but the feeling of not being protected enough there... ...perhaps the experience that protection was not sufficiently possible because no one was there to protect you or wanted to... ...because it happened that you were left alone in many situations in your life... ...and sometimes in life, you could have received help; it was perhaps within reach, but you no longer trusted and didn't want or couldn't take a risk anymore... ...That's how fear developed, and for you, it stayed as a fear of height, as a fear high up... ...because when you go up, climb a ladder, or an open staircase, it reminds you of situations of lacking protection... ...of lacking guidance when you needed guidance and help... ...But now you are there again and feel good because you are much stronger and more experienced than back then... ...You are here and today also in safety, and therefore you can endure the situation from back then well... ...perhaps back then it didn't even seem so dramatic to you, and the fear developed without you being able to recognize why... ...Today, everything is fine... ...and today, the past also relaxes because today, you have a different feeling about it... ...the calm feeling inside you that you now feel in the trance... ...That's good... ...You change your attitude towards the events back then... ...You free yourself from the fear of heights... ...This calm feeling you have now is the new feeling of the past and the new feeling of today...

And now hold onto this good feeling with your thoughts and prepare to travel through time with this relaxation... ...and on the return journey, you will experience the entire time of your life since then in just a few seconds, but today, this good feeling accompanies you through your life, a feeling completely without fear... ...Fear of heights cannot arise... ...You now travel through the time of your life and learn anew and differently from back then... ...You now learn, based on your good feeling, to build the new feeling of trust and security in connection with height... ...and when you arrive in the present, you feel safe even at heights... ...You return to the present... ...Now...

Hypnosis 10

I want to accompany you today on a very special inner journey... ...on a journey that takes place in your imagination... ...and at the same time in reality, in a very real and true world... ...because imagination is more than creative thinking or dreaming... ...Imagination is the liberated potential of our own creative power... ...Our imagination can create and dissolve worlds daily, creating new things and leading everything to a good end... ...But in all dreams and perhaps unimaginable images, there is always a special truth, a reality that always lies within our imagination and always shapes it... ...the truth of our feelings... ...because everything we can think of and dream about is an expression of our feelings... ...Imagination is, therefore, feeling turned into images... ...So, you go to that place in your imagination where your feelings turn into helpful images... ...into images that help you constructively change your life... ...You go to the land of dreams...

In the land of dreams, everything is as you want it... ...it looks like you like it... ...You can be by the sea and enjoy the sun, gaze out over the water or toward the horizon... ...or stand high on a mountain and overlook the entire land... ...enjoy the vastness and the height because in the land of dreams, you have no fear... ...it is the land of your imagination, and in your imagination, you have no fear... ...maybe in your waking life, you can't quite imagine being completely fearless, but in your imagination, you can... ...otherwise, you wouldn't be here, you wouldn't even try to get rid of the fear... ...So, you can imagine it... ...You could now imagine flying... ...in an airplane or on the back of a giant bird... ...or as a dragon rider... ...or standing on the roof of a skyscraper and finding it amusing; in your imagination, that's possible... ...but that's not what our journey is about... ...it's not about you intensely imagining being able to do that and being fearless... ...The land of dreams can do much more than that... ...You can do much more than that... ...You discover a staircase that goes from the ground up to the sky... ...It stands on a meadow and goes step by step into the sky... ...It goes so high up that you can't see the end; it's somewhere above the clouds... ...Maybe there's no end, and the staircase goes infinitely high and higher, who knows... ...You go to the staircase...

...It's wide, but there's no railing... ...Climbing it is easy in the land of dreams... ...But first, you simply go there... ...go to the staircase because there's a large sign in front of it with your name on it... ...You get closer because there's much more written on the sign... ...At the top, there's a heading, right under your name... ...It says: I fear heights because you know this feeling and want to understand it today... ...and understanding always means learning something new in the land of dreams... ...something that isn't really new but hasn't been seen yet... ...and thus, the fear dissolves... ...You keep looking at the sign, at this board on the staircase because underneath the heading are statements that you know... ...There are hints or comments there that you've heard often before or something similar... ...or they were never said out loud by anyone, but you had the impression that these expectations were placed on you... ...you were perhaps certain that these expectations were placed on you... ...Maybe it says there... ...Don't get too cocky... ...or... ...Pride comes before the fall... ...Maybe it says there: Don't make yourself bigger than others... ...or it even says there... ...You are worth nothing because you often had the feeling that your worth was not seen or recognized... ...maybe even early on, in your childhood... ...when you needed someone to tell you that you're good as you are... ...You needed someone to help you tell your wishes and dreams... ...but it was different... ...You often had the feeling that there was too little space for you and your ideas... ...or that no one could really understand you... ...You were once carefree as a child, but over the course of your life, you became more insecure... ...You remember... ...Over time, the fear arose that you could fall deeply if you became too big or too successful... ...You know the saying Pride comes before the fall... ...maybe you know the saying in English, which goes... ...The bigger they are, the harder they fall, which means that the bigger or more powerful we are, the harder we fall... ...But that wasn't your idea, and it was never your own fear... ...You felt it, you truly felt fear of and in height, but you carried it for others... ...You carried it for people for whom you limited yourself... ...for whom you stayed smaller than you actually wanted... ...It's not about a career, and it's not about financial success... ...it's about how you've often limited yourself in your self-development for others... ...maybe you wanted to comfort them or meet their expectations, just as you often met many expectations and put your own expectations of yourself on hold... ...And maybe on this sign, on the board at the staircase, there are other striking sentences or statements or expectations that you know well and can read there now... ...Then you think about how you've let yourself be limited for too long... ...and that you don't need to have fear of heights for others because this fear is a result of those old limits that you can't do anything about... ...You didn't choose them, but today you choose to leave those limits behind because the fear of heights was the feeling you carried for others... ...not for yourself, so you don't need it anymore... ...So, you go as fast as you can... ...You storm up the staircase, step by step, quickly, and you feel liberated doing it... ...You leave the sign of old expectations behind on the ground and run up the staircase into the sky of the dreamland... ...higher and higher with every step, and with each step you leave behind, you feel freer...

On your way to new freedom high above the clouds, you think about the land of dreams and how you can leave limits behind here, lift restrictions because in imagination, it's that simple... ...But the land of dreams is more than imagination... ...it exists... ...it lies deep within you and has always been there... ...I'm just telling you about it...

Distribution, publication, and copying in any form are prohibited and subject to damages.

All Titles in the Series

Volume 1: Smoking Cessation
Volume 2: Anxiety and Restlessness
Volume 3: Burnout
Volume 4: Reducing Overweight
Volume 5: Coping with the Past
Volume 6: Suicidal Thoughts and Attempts
Volume 7: Psycho-Oncology
Volume 8: Obsessions and Tics
Volume 9: Self-Confidence and Decision-Making
Volume 10: Grief Work
Volume 11: Psychosomatics
Volume 12: Chronic Pain
Volume 13: Depressive Thoughts
Volume 14: Panic Attacks
Volume 15: Domestic Violence, Victim Support
Volume 16: Post-Traumatic Stress
Volume 17: Exam Anxiety and Stage Fright
Volume 18: Anti-Violence Training, Offender Support
Volume 19: Addiction Tendencies
Volume 20: Social Phobia and Fear of Contact
Volume 21: Nail Biting
Volume 22: Self-Awareness and Self-Love
Volume 23: Teeth Grinding and Night Clenching
Volume 24: Feelings of Guilt
Volume 25: Fear in Crowds
Volume 26: Fear of Flying, Aviophobia
Volume 27: Fear in Enclosed Spaces, Claustrophobia
Volume 28: Tinnitus, Ear Noises
Volume 29: Fear of Heights
Volume 30: Neurodermatitis

Copying, publishing, and sharing with third parties are only permitted with the written consent of the author. Please observe the notes on copyright and usage.

- Volume 31: Finding Inner Balance
- Volume 32: Overcoming Loneliness
- Volume 33: Fear of Illness, Hypochondria
- Volume 34: Anticipatory Anxiety, Fear of Fear
- Volume 35: Jealousy in Relationships
- Volume 36: Driving Anxiety
- Volume 37: New Start after Separation
- Volume 38: Fear of Injections
- Volume 39: Heart Anxiety Neurosis
- Volume 40: Overcoming Resentment and Anger
- Volume 41: Resolving Blockages and Positive Thinking
- Volume 42: Stress Reduction, Stress Management
- Volume 43: Body Relaxation
- Volume 44: Deep Relaxation
- Volume 45: Fear of the Dark
- Volume 46: Falling Asleep and Staying Asleep
- Volume 47: Compulsive Buying
- Volume 48: Restless Legs Syndrome
- Volume 49: Bulimia
- Volume 50: Anorexia
- Volume 51: Overcoming Nightmares
- Volume 52: Imagined Deformity
- Volume 53: Overcoming Distrust, Finding Trust
- Volume 54: Processing Failures
- Volume 55: Humiliation, Emotional Hurt
- Volume 56: Distressing Compassion, Vicarious Suffering
- Volume 57: Self-Forgiveness
- Volume 58: Self-Awareness, Self-Confidence
- Volume 59: Saying No
- Volume 60: Assertiveness
- Volume 61: Setting Boundaries and Self-Assertion
- Volume 62: Decision-Making Ability

Volume 63: Success Orientation
Volume 64: Ruminating, Circular Thinking
Volume 65: Accepting Pregnancy
Volume 66: Birth Preparation
Volume 67: Spiritual Opening
Volume 68: Joy of Life and Inner Lightness
Volume 69: Patience and Inner Peace
Volume 70: Fibromyalgia and Rheumatism
Volume 71: Irritable Bowel Syndrome, Crohn's Disease
Volume 72: Fear of Nausea, Emetophobia
Volume 73: Stuttering and Cluttering, Speech Flow Disorders
Volume 74: Concentration and Knowledge Anchoring
Volume 75: Vitality and Spontaneity
Volume 76: Searching for Meaning and Finding Goals
Volume 77: Life Crises, Life Events
Volume 78: Workaholism, Goal Obsession
Volume 79: Helper Syndrome, Helpless Helpers
Volume 80: Medication Abuse
Volume 81: Gambling Addiction
Volume 82: Internet Addiction, Smartphone Addiction
Volume 83: Hoarding Disorder, Compulsive Collecting
Volume 84: Conspiracy Thoughts, Overvalued Ideas
Volume 85: Fear of Operations and Treatments
Volume 86: Fear of Aging
Volume 87: Travel Anxiety
Volume 88: Anxiety When Urinating, Paruresis
Volume 89: Fear of Intimacy and Togetherness
Volume 90: Fear of Blushing
Volume 91: Coming Out in Homosexuality
Volume 92: Charisma Training
Volume 93: Migraines and Chronic Headaches
Volume 94: Overcoming Allergies, Bronchial Asthma

Volume 95: Normalizing Blood Pressure
Volume 96: Compulsive Perfectionism
Volume 97: Sports Hypnosis, Motivation
Volume 98: Sports Hypnosis, Performance Enhancement
Volume 99: Determination and Focus
Volume 100: Encountering the Inner Child
Volume 101: Cravings, Binge Eating
Volume 102: Stimulating Metabolism
Volume 103: Bipolar Mood Swings
Volume 104: Borderline, Identity Crises
Volume 105: Hypomania, Euphoria, Mania
Volume 106: Restlessness, Agitation
Volume 107: Nervous Breakdown
Volume 108: Adjustment Disorders
Volume 109: Self-Alienation, Depersonalization
Volume 110: Ending Self-Pity
Volume 111: Primary Gain of Illness
Volume 112: Secondary Gain of Illness
Volume 113: Bullying, Victim Support
Volume 114: Letting Go of Envy and Jealousy
Volume 115: Fear of Spiders, Arachnophobia
Volume 116: Fear of Dogs or Cats
Volume 117: Fear of Strangers, Xenophobia
Volume 118: Excessive Worries, Generalized Anxiety
Volume 119: Strengthening Sense of Responsibility
Volume 120: Unrequited Love, Heartache
Volume 121: Work-Life Balance
Volume 122: Letting Go of Unattainable Goals
Volume 123: Allowing and Accepting Help
Volume 124: Letting Go of Adult Children
Volume 125: Tourette Syndrome
Volume 126: Life Changes and New Starts

Volume 127: Accepting Life in a Wheelchair
Volume 128: Understanding and Overcoming Homesickness
Volume 129: Understanding and Overcoming Wanderlust
Volume 130: Dizziness, Meniere's Disease
Volume 131: Overcoming Aggression
Volume 132: Cutting and Self-Harm
Volume 133: Hair Pulling, Trichotillomania
Volume 134: Postpartum Depression
Volume 135: For Relatives of Dementia Patients
Volume 136: Self-Harm, Artificial Disorders
Volume 137: Activating Self-Healing Powers
Volume 138: Preventing Depression Relapse
Volume 139: Reactive Psychoses, Follow-Up
Volume 140: Obsessive Thoughts and Impulses
Volume 141: Compulsive Checking
Volume 142: Compulsive Counting, Symmetry Obsession
Volume 143: Compulsive Washing, Cleanliness Obsession
Volume 144: Compulsive Questioning
Volume 145: Dissociative Paralysis
Volume 146: Phantom Pain
Volume 147: Overcoming Complaining
Volume 148: Hay Fever, Pollen Allergy
Volume 149: Sexual Abuse, Victim Support
Volume 150: Standing Strong Against Sexism, #metoo
Volume 151: Binge Eating
Volume 152: Overcoming Thoughts of Revenge
Volume 153: Detachment from the Aggressor, Stockholm Syndrome
Volume 154: Courage to Separate
Volume 155: Chronic Fatigue, Exhaustion
Volume 156: Fear of the Future, Existential Anxiety
Volume 157: Excessive Worry About Children
Volume 158: Fear of Failure

Volume 159: Ending Distrust and Control
Volume 160: Dejection, Dysphoria
Volume 161: Boreout, Chronic Boredom
Volume 162: Bipolar Disorders, Relapse Prevention
Volume 163: Mania, Relapse Prevention
Volume 164: Nihilism, Feelings of Worthlessness
Volume 165: Thumb Sucking
Volume 166: Being Brave
Volume 167: Being Proud
Volume 168: Overcoming Shyness
Volume 169: Being Able to Delegate Responsibility
Volume 170: Being Able to Show Emotions
Volume 171: Letting Go of Guilt, Victim Support
Volume 172: Processing Guilt, Offender Support
Volume 173: Mood Swings, Cyclothymia
Volume 174: Lack of Drive, Vital Sadness
Volume 175: Hearing Voices with Reality Reference
Volume 176: Confident Communication
Volume 177: Standing Up for Oneself
Volume 178: Taking New Paths
Volume 179: Confident Job Application
Volume 180: No Longer Being Taken Advantage Of
Volume 181: End of Submissiveness
Volume 182: Depressive Numbness
Volume 183: Mood Drops, Affective Incontinence
Volume 184: Mood Instability
Volume 185: Somatoform Disorders
Volume 186: Stomach Ulcer, Psychosomatic
Volume 187: Accepting Amputation
Volume 188: Overcoming and Letting Go of Hatred
Volume 189: Ending Accusations
Volume 190: Allowing Tears, Being Able to Cry

Volume 191: Finding and Sorting Repressed Feelings
Volume 192: Somatoform Pain
Volume 193: Living Autonomously
Volume 194: Anhedonia, Joylessness
Volume 195: Persistent Sadness
Volume 196: Obesity, Food Addiction
Volume 197: Parents of Abused Children
Volume 198: Letting Go and Letting Be
Volume 199: Childhood Sexual Abuse
Volume 200: Fear of Loss